The Next Medical
REVOLUTION

ANGIOLOGY

Prevent your
Heart Attack or Stroke

The Next Medical
REVOLUTION

ANGIOLOGY

Prevent your
Heart Attack or Stroke

A. S. Callahan III MD

ALTMAN

Published by Altman Publishing Ltd, 7 Ash Copse, Bricket Wood, St Albans, Hertfordshire AL2 3YA, England
info@altman-publishing.com

First edition 2004
Reprinted 2005

The rights of A. S. Callahan III to be identified as the Author of this Work have been asserted by him in accordance with the Copyright, Designs and Patents Act 1988.

Typeset in 10/12.5 Optima by Scribe Design, Gillingham, Kent, England
Printed in the United States of America by BookMaster, Inc., Mansfield, Ohio

ISBN 1 86036 029 7

The publisher makes no representation, express or implied, with regard to the accuracy of the information contained in this book and cannot accept any legal responsibility or liability for any errors or omissions that may be made.

Library of Congress
Cataloging-in-Publication Data has been applied for

British Library
Cataloguing-in-Publication Data has been applied for

CONTENTS

Dedicated to Barbara Massey Rogers

PREFACE

Sometimes a chance encounter or event can shape an entire book. The catalyst for this book was a Danish fence. An outstanding Danish vascular surgeon and friend, Dr Henrik Sillesen, showed me around his garden one spring afternoon. Separating his house from the adjacent ones was an unpainted wooden fence. The slats were arranged horizontally, so that each piece ran from the outside of one post to the inside of the next. When I asked about this design, his reply provided a parable for integrated vascular care. He said:

> Fences here are different than in America. You put fence slats on vertically, so when an area rots away at the bottom, all must be replaced. With our arrangement we only have to replace a single bottom slat. Your fences have their nice side on only one side. With our construction the fence looks the same on my neighbor's side as it does on my side – we both have a nice view.

Dr Sillesen's explanation of the fence construction also illuminated differences in vascular care between his country and mine. For him, being parsimonious with resources was significant, rather than being wasteful with the wood. Further, he looked after his neighbor as himself. Both had an equally pleasing view. In contrast, American vascular care is fragmented. Because it is procedurally based, it is very expensive and wasteful of resources. The care that we give is not the same for all our neighbors as it is for ourselves. Unequal access to care is an issue in the United States.

Despite the American egocentric view of healthcare, many medical advances are not routinely made available to patients. We spend more and do more but whether we provide greater benefits is uncertain. This book provides the reader an insider view of vascular healthcare, and hopefully dismisses some unnecessary mystery from medicine.

Readers who are concerned about their vascular health can readily access information about integrated vascular care – the vascular care of the future. Our vascular destinies are the sum of many small decisions made years ago. Tomorrow starts yesterday. This book seeks to provide you with medical information that can inform your healthcare decisions in the future. Armed with these facts, you will be ready to participate in the coming revolution in vascular medical care: the angiology way.

INTRODUCTION

Heart disease is the leading cause of death in the United States and in other industrialized nations. In 2000, there were nearly 2.5 million deaths from all causes in the USA, and nearly one-third of these were from heart disease. The third leading cause of death was stroke, so that heart disease and stroke together killed nearly 900,000 people in that one year, the latest for which statistics are available. That works out at 100 people every hour every day. Put another way, in the United States there is a stroke every 50 seconds and a heart attack every 30 seconds.

The sad thing about these events is that many of them are preventable by lifestyle changes and proper medication. That's what this book is about – how to change your vascular destiny. Don't become a casualty before the coming revolution in vascular care benefits you.

1   THE PROBLEM – WHAT CAUSES HEART ATTACKS AND STROKES?

The seeds of a heart attack or stroke are sown many years before they happen. While these events occur suddenly and at times without warning, their occurrence is pre-ordained by the hardening and narrowing of the arteries – atherosclerosis, a process that actually begins during our teenage years. When heart transplantation took off in the late 1960s, doctors were able to examine the hearts of many young people who had died in road traffic and other accidents, and it became clear that hardening of the arteries occurred at a much younger age than had previously been thought. Nearly 17% of people under the age of 20 had clogged arteries. By the age of 40, more than half of us will have such changes in our blood vessels.

The sheer number of heart attacks and strokes is impressive. There are about 1 million heart attacks each year and nearly 750,000 strokes (see Figures 1.1, 1.2). About half of these heart attacks are fatal, although there are, of course, millions of Americans who have had heart attacks and strokes who survive.

Heart attack and stroke are the first and third leading causes of death for Americans. Of the 1 million heart attacks that happen each year,

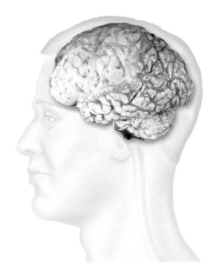

Figure 1.1   Side view of left side of the brain with stroke.

Stroke   Stroke

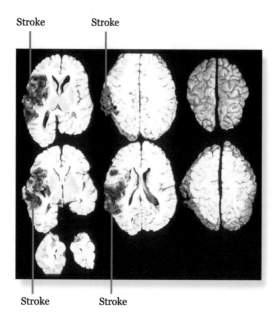

Figure 1.2 Sliced left side of the brain with stroke.

Stroke   Stroke

about one-third are first heart attacks and the rest are repeat attacks. The significant occurrence of heart attacks and strokes makes it a public health issue. The annual direct expense represented by heart attack and stroke combined is more than US$300 billion. However, the impact of these two illnesses is far greater than any dollar measure. An individual's life is rarely the same after suffering either a heart attack or a stroke. Stroke is the leading cause of adult disability, so, while it is not always fatal, it is often ruinous.

In the past it was thought that the hardening and narrowing of our blood vessels was a process that proceeded in a somewhat regular manner over time. The older we got, the narrower our blood vessels became. The underlying assumption was that very narrowed arteries caused heart attacks and strokes. Known risk factors such as high blood pressure, diabetes, smoking, obesity, sedentary lifestyle, high cholesterol, and genes were felt to be accelerators of this progressive change in our blood vessels.

Such a simple view of gradual narrowing led to new means of enlarging blocked blood vessels or bypassing them to increase blood flow. Balloon angioplasty (passing a tube into the blocked vessel and using it to inflate a small balloon to widen the vessel), and surgical bypass (grafting an unblocked blood vessel, say from the patient's leg, to enable the blood to flow around the obstruction) were developed. Since most people have narrowed blood vessels, millions of these procedures are performed in the United States each year. As our population ages, there is likely to be a steady increase in the number of such procedures. Increased expenditures for these operations will spark debate about financing healthcare for patients with blockages. This entire debate is based on the assumption that blood vessels undergo a gradual and progressive narrowing with age.

When young patients who died of heart attacks had their coronary arteries studied, two-thirds of them had narrowing that was LESS than half of the artery's diameter, and only about 15% had narrowing MORE than three-quarters of the artery's diameter. So, the **MORE** narrowed arteries caused **FEWER** fatal heart attacks than the **LESS** narrow ones. This observation suggested that the **type** of narrowing was the important factor, rather than the **amount** of narrowing.

Hardening of the arteries is due to a build-up of materials in the blood vessel – this mass of materials is called a plaque. This plaque has an inner core and an outside lining or cap. Studies of fatal heart attacks in young people revealed that despite having only slight narrowing, plaques had ruptured and their outside lining had been torn. When a plaque that produced only slight narrowing ruptured in this way, circulating blood cells would come in contact with the ruptured plaque and produce a local blood clot over the plaque surface. This clot might completely block the artery – something that the plaque had not done – or it might be swept away and travel into downstream blood vessels where it could create a blockage.

The realization that the cause of heart attacks and strokes was plaque rupture rather than artery narrowing would dictate a different approach to disease prevention. Instead of trying to open up blood vessels, one would try to keep the plaques from rupturing. Strategies for doing this might include keeping a thick or firm outer lining and/or reducing the inner core of the plaque. Such a program would seek to keep plaque STABLE and to try to prevent it from becoming UNSTABLE (see Figures 1.3, 1.4).

Once the focus shifted from relief of blockage to changing the character of the blocking plaque, different strategies for medical management came into being. Such management would attempt to keep plaque stable and to live with the degree of narrowing that is present. Since the narrowing process is so common and heart attacks and strokes are less common, it is clear that most of us are living with blockages. What we seek is a way to keep our blockages from causing a heart attack or stroke.

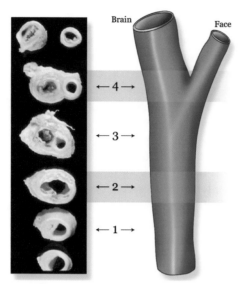

Figure 1.3 Left carotid artery that caused stroke.

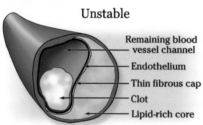

Unstable

Remaining blood vessel channel
Endothelium
Thin fibrous cap
Clot
Lipid-rich core

Figure 1.4 Stable and unstable plaque. (Endothelium – the inside lining cells of blood vessels. This lining separates flowing blood from the plaque or middle and outer parts of the blood vessel.)

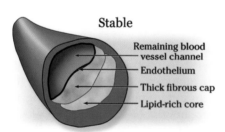

Stable

Remaining blood vessel channel
Endothelium
Thick fibrous cap
Lipid-rich core

If there were a way to identify which blockages were unstable, then we could monitor medical therapy. We could utilize alternative means of dealing with the plaque, using balloons or surgery only when necessary. Specialized medical programs exist to help stabilize vulnerable plaque. Personal initiatives for activity can enhance such programs and provide incremental benefits.

The advent of non-invasive therapies for plaque stabilization depended on the identification of plaque rupture rather than progressive narrowing as the main cause of heart attacks and strokes. Identifying both the presence of arterial narrowing and its specific features is necessary to plan a program of intervention. Such detailed knowledge of the plaque would result in fewer operations with balloons or plaque removal. An ensemble approach including personal initiatives plus medications could be highly beneficial, resulting in a reduced financial burden for the aging population as well. A clearer understanding of these challenges permits preventive measures.

Once vulnerable plaque has become unstable or "hot" a person is at risk for a heart attack or stroke. If sufficient backup blood flows past the blocked artery, through another artery, a person might exhibit minimal clinical symptoms of a heart attack or stroke or none at all. In response to gradual narrowing of the arteries, the body tries to improve its backup blood supply. However, when vulnerable plaque becomes unstable and there is inadequate backup blood flow, then the clinical consequences are more likely to be severe.

The vulnerable plaque that has become unstable confers RISK of a heart attack or stroke. Yet the risk that is created is not constant. Once the plaque is unstable it does not always remain unstable. It is possible for the unstable plaque to become stable again, although this does not always happen.

There are four arteries that supply the brain with blood, two each in the front and back, two each on the right and left. The front arteries are called the carotid arteries and the ones that go to the brain are called the internal carotid arteries. The back arteries are called vertebral arteries and in the skull they join to form a single artery. This is the only spot in the body where two arteries become one. Normally each artery divides into two and those subdivide into another two, much like tree limbs. Presumably the reason for having two of each artery is to provide for a backup in case of trouble.

When carotid arteries narrow, they can produce strokes involving the front of the brain. Narrowings in these arteries can reduce blood flow, making the resulting flow noisy or turbulent. Since the carotid arteries run towards the brain in the neck, it is possible to study them with Doppler or ultrasound devices. An arteriogram or angiogram procedure can produce an x-ray movie of the flowing blood in the carotid arteries. The resulting pictures show the plaque that is present in the arteries. Identification of significant blockage often leads to surgical removal of the plaque, a procedure called endarterectomy. In the United States there are about 150,000 such carotid cleanout procedures performed annually. This cleanout procedure was developed in the early 1950s, but it was not until the 1990s that the procedure was proven to prevent strokes.

The study of the surgical cleanout was called **N**orth **A**merican **S**ymptomatic **C**arotid **E**ndarterectomy **T**rial, normally abbreviated as NASCET. This study used the results of the angiogram pictures to measure the amount of narrowing in the carotid arteries. Among patients with more than 70% narrowing, those who underwent endarterectomy experienced reduced risk of stroke when compared to patients who were given medication alone.

The risk of carotid stroke was higher when narrowing exceeded 70%. In NASCET all the narrowed arteries were considered symptomatic, suggesting that the visible plaque had become unstable. At the conclusion of the trial, most patients taking medication continued to do so rather than have surgery. Over the next 2.5 years, strokes continued to occur in the medication-only group at a rate higher than those patients who had surgery. However, after 2.5 years there was NO difference in the stroke rate or risk between those who were taking medications and those who had surgery. The lack of further enhanced risk continued over the next 3.5 years of follow-up (see Figure 1.5).

In other words, the risk of stroke from an unstable carotid plaque seemed to last 2.5 years. After that period of time, while the artery was still just as narrow as before, it no longer seemed to confer any risk. Thirty percent of patients receiving medication experienced a stroke over the 2.5 years, while 70% did not. The natural history of the

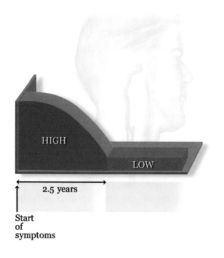

Figure 1.5 Risk of stroke from unstable carotid plaque.

HIGH

LOW

2.5 years

Start
of
symptoms

unstable carotid plaque was that only the minority of patients was at risk. This study suggested that there were forces at work that could modify or change unstable plaque and make it stable again. Apparently, within 2.5 years the body or natural forces stabilized the plaque. Arteries that were diseased seemed to be able to heal. Knowing that such healing is possible, it seems reasonable to consider how to accelerate or positively influence this healing process.

The tears that occur when unstable plaque is vulnerable and become critically ruptured can also occur in normal arteries. Such tears are called dissections and often occur when a normal artery gets sharply impacted by a nearby bone during trauma. At times the trauma can seem to be trivial, such as during a sneeze or when bending the neck for a long period of time. Sometime the trauma is unidentified. The exaggerated body movements necessary to produce such dissections normally occur in young people.

Case study 1

Linda is a healthy young woman who has developed a business that specializes in beauty products. Because of her business success, a leading woman's magazine wanted to feature her story and scheduled an interview in New York City. The interview was intense and lasted more than 2 hours. As Linda left midtown Manhattan, she decided to walk up 5th Avenue to shop. After walking several of the short blocks at her usual brisk pace, her right eye became suddenly blind. The vision in this eye seemed to be foggy (gray cloud of mist) or like looking through a heavy rain at night. She had no other symptoms and continued walking. Within a minute or two her vision had completely returned to normal.

The next morning when Linda awoke and got out of bed, her right eye again became blind in exactly the same fashion. Her right eyelid seemed to be drooping and she experienced a new pain like a vague ache over her right eyebrow. Though the visual loss was again temporary, lasting only a few minutes, the ache did not stop. When Linda again had visual loss while working out with her personal trainer, she decided to speak with her physician. Several tests confirmed that her right internal carotid artery was completely blocked in the neck (see Figure 1.6). The blockage was not due to hardening of the arteries but was due to a tear in the artery just where it enters the skull.

Linda had no risk factors for stroke. She had no history of smoking, hypertension, diabetes or high cholesterol. She was not overweight and participated in a regular exercise program. Despite the lack of risk

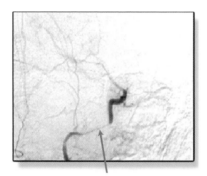 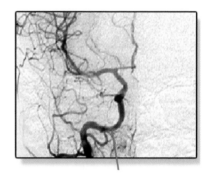

Figure 1.6 Carotid dissection (arrow) at symptom onset.

Figure 1.7 Carotid dissection (arrow) 15 months later (normal carotid artery).

factors and a lifestyle thought to lower risk of stroke and heart attack, she had a completely blocked internal carotid artery. Her symptoms mimicked a stroke.

Serial studies over the next 15 months confirmed that the artery that had been completely blocked had then returned to a completely normal condition (see Figure 1.7). Linda was indeed fortunate.

Identification of the dissection (tear) of a normal blood vessel permitted medical therapy to prevent a stroke during the vulnerable window while the artery was healing. The body is able to heal tears in normal blood vessels and it can also heal tears in diseased ones. And tearing is what makes vulnerable plaques become unstable, producing clotting and perhaps a heart attack or stroke. Tears take between 1.5 and 2.5 years to heal – a lot of time. The issue then is how to get time on our side.

Summary

- Heart attacks and strokes occur when blockages in arteries become UNSTABLE, not just narrow.
- Most heart attacks occur in arteries that have only mild narrowing.
- It is important to know the nature of the narrowing in our arteries, not just how narrow.
- Unstable plaques create RISK which declines over time – this risk can be modified by medication and personal initiatives.
- Unstable plaque causes a heart attack or stroke when the plaque tears or dissects. Such tears can HEAL as is known to occur with dissections in normal blood vessel walls.

2 CHOLESTEROL – WHAT IS IT AND WHY IS IT IMPORTANT?

Cholesterol is a fatty substance present in many animal and dairy products and also produced naturally by the liver. It is needed by the body as it is used in the production of steroid hormones and other important materials that are required to keep us healthy. However, too much of it has been found to be a bad thing. How did this finding come about? It is a long, and sometimes complicated, story but worth knowing. However, before embarking on that, we need to explain briefly how cholesterol is carried around in the blood and how much of it we really need.

Most of the cholesterol in the blood is carried around attached to protein molecules. There are two types, called **low density lipoprotein (LDL)** and **high density lipoprotein (HDL)**. We therefore speak of LDL-cholesterol and HDL-cholesterol. About 70% of the cholesterol in the blood is carried around as LDL-cholesterol with the remaining 30% being HDL-cholesterol. It turns out that the HDL protein is involved in removing excess cholesterol from the blood, thus preventing its build-up in the arteries. This has resulted in HDL-cholesterol being referred to as good cholesterol and a higher value is better than a lower value (see Table 2.1). Conversely, the LDL protein carries the cholesterol to the cells in the body's organs, so that LDL-cholesterol is referred to as

Table 2.1 Desirable values for blood cholesterol levels (mg/dL)
(Figures in white are in units of mmol/L as used in the UK and some other countries).

Cholesterol type	Value		Comment
Total cholesterol			
Desirable	< 200	< 5.2	
Borderline	200–240	5.2–6.2	
High	> 240	> 6.2	
LDL-cholesterol ('bad' cholesterol)			
Desirable	< 100	< 2.6	
Borderline	100–160	2.6–4.2	
High	> 160	> 4.2	HIGH RISK!!
HDL-cholesterol ('good' cholesterol)			
Low	< 40	< 1.0	HIGH RISK!!
Desirable	> 50	> 1.3	

bad cholesterol, as a high value is bad. Your LDL-cholesterol level is a good indicator of your risk for heart disease, and the main aim of any treatment is to lower the LDL-cholesterol level.

When too much LDL-cholesterol circulates in the blood, it can slowly build up in the walls of the arteries that feed the heart and brain and contribute to forming the plaques that were described in Chapter 1.

Doctors sometimes use the ratio of total cholesterol to HDL-cholesterol as an indicator of your risk of developing heart disease or stroke. The optimum value for the ratio is less than 5:1. A value of between 3:1 and 4:1 would be desirable.

Having gone into some detail about cholesterol, how it is carried around in the blood, and what current medical opinion is about desirable levels, let's now return to the story of how all this information was obtained.

With a mounting epidemic of cardiovascular disease beginning in the 1930s, the United States Public Health Service decided to undertake a large-scale study to investigate why heart disease had become the nation's number one killer by the late 1940s. Researchers wanted to learn which biological and environmental factors were contributing to such a rapid rise in cardiovascular death. They settled on a population-based study designed to learn how and why those who developed heart disease differed from those who escaped it.

Such a study would require many years of observation of a well-defined group of people. A thorough investigation of the people at the start of the study would give detailed information of their lifestyle and state of health so that this information could eventually be correlated when, many years later, some of these people suffered heart attacks and strokes. The small town of Framingham, 18 miles west of Boston, became the site for one of the most famous and far-reaching medical studies ever conducted. Framingham was chosen partly because it had a very stable population, so that there was a good chance that the same people would be available for continuous study over many years. In 1948, 740 volunteers were recruited, and eventually 5,209 healthy people aged between 30 and 60 were recruited from the town's population of 28,000. In 1971, the study recruited 5,124 children (and their spouses) of the original 5,209 for a second study, the "Offspring Study." With two generations worth of data, the Framingham Heart Study acquired an unmatched base of scientific riches.

This remarkable study has so far lasted for over 50 years and data are still being collected. It is one of the most important studies in the history of American, and probably world, medicine.

Before Framingham, most physicians believed that narrowing and hardening of the arteries was an inevitable part of the aging process and that blood pressure was supposed to increase with age so that the heart was better equipped to pump blood through an elderly person's narrowed arteries. The notion that scientists could identify and individuals could modify **risk factors** tied to heart disease, stroke and other diseases, was not part of standard medical practice. The majority of physicians did not understand the relationship, for example, between high levels of cholesterol and heart attacks. Many did not believe that modifying certain behaviors could enable their patients to avoid or reverse the underlying causes of serious heart and vascular conditions. Today, managing cholesterol levels, high blood pressure and diabetes to mitigate heart and vascular disease and stroke is fundamental to good medical care.

As the study began, 45% of the participants had total cholesterol levels of more than 240 mg/dL (milligrams per deciliter, the units in which cholesterol is measured in the blood). This was the older upper limit of what was considered normal. Excluding participants under 45 years of age, women comprised the majority of those with elevated cholesterol. After 16 years of follow-up there had been 193 heart attacks out of 1,571 men. Of men who entered the study with a total cholesterol greater than 320, **ALL** had had a heart attack after 16 years. Among men who entered the study with a total cholesterol below 150, **NONE** had had a heart attack after 16 years.

After 26 years of study, all men who began the study with a total cholesterol of greater than 300 had had a heart attack. Those with cholesterol levels below 150 had not had a heart attack. Over time, then, more of the men with higher cholesterols were having heart attacks. Yet by 26 years, 35% of those who had heart attacks had enrollment cholesterols below 200 (the **NEW** upper limit of normal). So a "normal" level of cholesterol did not mean things were all right or that you were safe from a heart attack (see Figure 2.1).

Because high cholesterols were associated with heart attacks in men and low levels were not, the lipid hypothesis was developed. Since high levels of cholesterol were associated with risk of heart attacks, it seemed that cholesterol must have something to do with hardening of the arteries. While the hypothesis was borne out at the high and low levels of blood cholesterol, in the middle there was overlap between the presence or absence of heart attacks. So the lipid hypothesis had great predictive power at the very high and very low levels. But in between it could not predict who would or would not have a heart attack. For this in-between

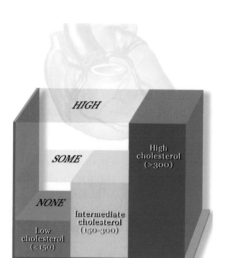

Figure 2.1   Risk of heart attack.

group there was only a percentage of risk and an individual would not know which group he was in before a heart attack occurred.

One means of proving the lipid hypothesis would be to lower the cholesterol level in a group of individuals and see if they had fewer heart attacks than those without this reduction. The advent of **statins**, a group of drugs that have a remarkable ability to lower cholesterol, permitted such studies. In all the various clinical trials with each of the available statins, there was a roughly 30% reduction in heart attacks for those patients who received this cholesterol-lowering medication.

The association of lower cholesterol levels with lower risk of heart attack seemed to validate the lipid hypothesis. A lower cholesterol level appeared better than a higher one and the benefit from taking statins seemed to be associated with lowering the cholesterol level. Now it would be important to see if the lipid hypothesis had utility in patients with stroke.

Cholesterol levels have a different association with stroke than that identified with heart attacks in the Framingham study. Very low cholesterol levels in the blood have been associated with bleeding in the brain (called hemorrhagic stroke). However, over a very broad range of cholesterol levels from about 180 to 260, studies have NOT shown an association of cholesterol level with stroke (ischemic or non-bleeding stroke). The finding that cholesterol levels would have an association with heart disease and not with stroke is a paradox that has not been explained completely.

This paradox of the contrast in heart disease as opposed to stroke has been further intensified by studies of heart attack patients taking statins demonstrating a reduction in stroke frequency. Why should taking a cholesterol-lowering drug reduce the incidence of strokes in patients who have had heart attacks? If the lipid hypothesis has a very poor fit for stroke, then why would lipid lowering by statins provide any reduction of stroke in cardiac patients who have moderate to high levels of LDL- (bad) cholesterol?

Insight into these unexpected findings has come from studies of patients who did not have a history of heart attacks and who were studied BEFORE any problem occurred. The patients who were given a statin will have their cholesterol lowered. It is possible to match these patients with those who are not taking any statins. The overlap group can then be monitored for occurrence of heart attacks. When this was done in a Scottish trial, 2,191 men comprised the overlap. The men taking statins had 67 heart attacks while those who had the **same cholesterol level** but were not taking statins had 108 heart attacks. The inevitable conclusion was that the cholesterol-lowering medication was doing something more than just lowering the cholesterol. Some of the benefit of the drug was NOT related to cholesterol lowering. So, if we consider two people with the **same cholesterol level**, one being the natural level in the body without any medication, and the other being the result of taking a statin drug, then the person who is taking the statin will have a LOWER RISK of having a heart attack. That was a very surprising discovery.

The ability of statins to reduce stroke risk and confer more benefit than just cholesterol lowering suggests a non-cholesterol effect is at work in patients with vascular disease. In order to develop better means of assessing personal vascular risks, we must focus on more than just cholesterol levels. We therefore need to approach the problem of hardening of the arteries with techniques that indicate more precise risk. Directly visualizing plaque and its components may permit better identification of those at risk for heart attack and stroke. Therapies for risk reduction have their greatest benefit when used by persons with highest risk.

Summary

- Cholesterol levels are only personally predictive when low or high. Mid-range values do not indicate whether you will have a heart attack or stroke.
- Cholesterol-lowering medications, the statins, reduce heart attack risk by means other than lowering cholesterol levels. The statins then have NON-CHOLESTEROL EFFECTS.

3 EARLY WARNINGS – WHAT TO DO

When arteries are narrowed by plaque, activated or "hot" plaque may shed debris and cause temporary obstruction. Symptoms may develop that constitute a warning that more permanent problems or conditions could occur. Such an event in one of the arteries of the heart is called **angina**, and manifests itself as a chest pain. When it occurs in one of the arteries that go to the brain, it is called **TIA** or **transient ischemic attack**. TIA should also mean **take immediate action**. It is important to recognize these warnings in order to prevent a heart attack or stroke. To neglect the warnings is to lose the chance to see if one's vascular fate or future might be changed.

Case study 2

Don was visiting Santa Fe, New Mexico, when he noted that walking the town square made him short-winded. Despite slowing down and bidding his companions to go along, he noted that he was unable to keep up with his friends. When he sat down, his breath and energy gradually returned. He had not noted such symptoms when he had been walking at much lower elevations (Santa Fe is at 6000 feet above sea level). Despite the fact that he had suffered a stroke several years earlier, he did not seek medical help, even after his return home. Once home he noted that he was not so short-winded, but he did not seem to have the exercise tolerance that he had before the trip.

When he finally did seek medical help, tests revealed that he had more than 80% blockage of the left main coronary artery – also known as the **widow maker**. After re-vascularization by surgical means, he noted an immediate increase in his exercise tolerance. Because his tolerance had gradually diminished, the decline had been imperceptible. Once the decline was evident, he ascribed the new symptoms to having not been sufficiently active in the recent past. Explaining new symptoms due to pre-existing conditions is common. On the face of it, something new may be NEW and not a different manifestation of something old.

More often there can be chest pain that occurs occasionally but is not sharp. Such pain is usually provoked by exertion or exercise. The character of the pain is a pressure-type discomfort, which may be accompanied by sweating, shortness of breath and a change of skin color. The pain often occurs in sites other than the chest – involvement of the arm (often left), jaw or neck may occur.

Case study 3

Tracy, a nurse, was watching her grandson perform in a local production of Oklahoma! when she noted that her left upper lip was numb. She described this sensation as very unusual, like going to the dentist and getting a shot of novocaine. The numbness lasted about a minute or so. There was no other symptom at that time. Before the end of the show, the very same symptoms had recurred. After returning home she took an aspirin and smoked a cigarette.

Tracy had no history of high blood pressure, high cholesterol, heart disease or diabetes. Her mother had told her that she was invincible and she felt that most of us think we are, and that "these are minor irritations that are going to go away." However, her maternal grandmother had a stroke in her 70s.

When recurring episodes were measured, they lasted 3.5 minutes. During one of the episodes it was clear that her speech was effortful and thick-tongued although she could walk on her toes and heels with no imbalance or weakness. When the spell was over, she was completely normal.

Two days after the onset of the spells of left lip numbness, Tracy again experienced numbness during church. It spread into the palate and there was a problem with swallowing. Despite being a stroke nurse for years, "Not once did it cross my mind that I was having a stroke." She had as many as 20 episodes over the first 3 days.

Severe blockage of the right internal carotid artery was identified by studies and surgical cleanout was recommended. Before having the surgery performed, she left the hospital to go home and shampoo her hair. After her shower she returned to the hospital and was admitted for the operation. Her leisurely approach to threatening stroke was noteworthy.

After the procedure she had a different perspective:

First of all don't follow my example of self-diagnosis and delay. That is something most of us tend to do. Listen to your body. Pay close attention and get in touch with your physician. As a nurse working in rehabilitation, I jokingly said I might have to do my own evaluation for admission (to stroke rehab). I want to reiterate to individuals out there NOT to delay calling their physicians when symptoms occur. If you don't know what it is or you are afraid of sounding foolish – forget those things. Go ahead and call. Get help.

A TIA represents a small version of what a coming stroke would be. Usually symptoms recur, are always the same, are brief and occur without warning. When the symptoms last longer than 5 minutes, then probably a small stroke rather than a warning has occurred.

When the front of the brain's circulation is impaired, the symptoms will be numbness and/or weakness of the face, arm or combination, and loss of vision in a single eye. Speech may be involved if the blockage is in an artery going to the left side of the brain. If the back of the brain's circulation is involved, the symptoms will be different since different brain functions occur in the back of the brain.

Case study 4

Charles reported:

I started having brief, sudden headaches that would localize to the left rear quadrant of my head and my vision would blur. I would take three to four ibuprofen-type drugs and the pain would go away after I lay down. This had happened for several days. On Thursday I diagnosed myself as having a vision problem, so I went to see my ophthalmologist and explained my symptoms. You may remember that several years ago we joked about frying our brains with cell phones and he made a joke about my having done just that. He gave me a prescription for new glasses. On Saturday I went flying in a sail plane with my son. We did mild aerobatics, steep turns, some figure eights, nothing more than 2 G of force. By the time we landed I had a severe headache. It was such a severe headache that my son drove home. I just felt sick and didn't want to be bothered with driving and my vision was messed up. These symptoms had come and gone over a period of 3 weeks, but the episode after the sail plane persisted. The next morning I rose from bed and the headache came again, along with blurred vision. Nausea began and I lost my balance. My symptoms that day were the same as before but more intense. That morning I lost my balance and was unable to walk the hallway at home. I made it to the bathroom where I collapsed.

The combination of visual change and imbalance suggests that the blocked artery is one of those that go to the rear of the brain. These warning symptoms may last longer than those from the front arteries. Headache can be a symptom that accompanies blockages in the rear of the brain. Dizziness is the most vexing symptom to evaluate for importance.

Often when there is dizziness and numbness, paralysis, blurred or double vision, and speech impairment, the problem is circulatory. This is called **dizziness plus**. However, when dizziness occurs alone, there is uncertainty about what the symptom might indicate.

Case study 5

Yuri, a 35-year-old religious immigrant from Russia, tells it best:

I thought I was the healthiest man in the world. I had quit smoking a long time ago and I played tennis every other day. For a couple of days while I was at work, I felt a little dizziness, a little strange, thinking what is this? It happened for a few seconds, some kind of bad feeling to which I didn't pay attention. Very quickly it was gone – I thought that it was some kind of allergy. If you had mentioned to me that it was a stroke, then I would have laughed in your face.

On Monday morning about 6 o'clock I woke up and felt bad. I went to the bathroom and looked into the mirror seeing myself and at the same time getting blind. I couldn't feel on my left. I had to do something but I didn't know what. I fell down and couldn't raise my legs or my hand and then I started to throw up. I told my wife call the ambulance; I thought that I was going to die.

The first question the emergency personnel asked was had I been drinking? In the ER the first doctor said that it looked like an ear infection and that I was too young to have a stroke. Yet they were wrong. It is difficult to think that my life was over – at just 35. No one in my family had ever had a stroke. So I would say than I am Christopher Columbus. I was the first.

Dizziness plus blindness and paralysis is **NEVER** from the inner ear – it is always vascular insufficiency in the brain's back arteries.

TIA episodes are exactly the same. The clots that are created over activated plaque travel to the same destination within the brain and so the same territory of the body is affected by lack of function. The occurrence of TIAs means that the plaque has become unstable or "hot" and the episodes continue until the plaque becomes quiescent or a stroke occurs. Because of the long time necessary for the plaque to become quiet again, one can expect more TIAs or perhaps the next one might be the stroke. So urgent evaluation and treatment is warranted – which is why we say that TIA means **take immediate action**.

When you seek medical help, you have to be careful to seek the correct help. Glasses will not fix a circulatory problem in the arteries that go to the brain. So when symptoms are so novel and unusual, you should not accept being dismissed from the medical system with a routine or mundane suggestion. TIAs can occur in perfectly healthy people, who may have no risk factors for stroke and who are young. You can't diagnose yourself – even medical people get it wrong – and there should be no comfort in the fact that the episode was short and went away. The very nature of a TIA is that it is brief – the blockage is brief or the debris is small and the body is able to dissolve it quickly. Once a TIA is over you are still normal as you were before.

So pay attention and take action. Once these warnings occur, you have been served notice that the hardening of your arteries has progressed to unstable plaque. In order to prevent either a stroke or a heart attack you will need to adopt a more aggressive program of vascular care.

Summary

- Angina is an early warning symptom of coronary insufficiency. It is defined as chest tightness or pressure, often with an ache in either arm (often the left) or jaw ache in concert with exertion.
- TIAs are warnings of an impending stroke. These sudden, temporary and stereotypic spells (they are always the same) include difficulty speaking, imbalance, numbness to one side of the body (often face and arm or face/arm/leg), weakness to one side of the body (often face and arm or face/arm/leg), blindness in one eye, double vision. These generally last only 5 minutes or less.

4   REDUCING RISK – LIFESTYLE CHANGES

Because hardening of the arteries is so common and event rates for heart attacks and stroke are so high, it is natural to search for programs of action that will reduce risk or change one's vascular fate. Such programs would include a central core of cost-effective interventions and personally chosen health strategies.

One such cost-effective, personal strategy is the decision not to smoke. The ability of blood vessels to repair themselves is negatively influenced by smoking. Smoke inhalation exposes the blood vessels to the absorbed products of combustion along with nicotine. Even the use of smokeless tobacco results in the absorption of chemicals into the bloodstream through the mouth. This contact with foreign chemicals interferes with the ability of the lining cells of the artery wall to function properly. Stopping smoking or never beginning the habit is a powerful way to lower one's vascular risk.

We can choose to use our time in ways that may modify vascular risk. Generally time would not be considered an ally since vascular risk increases with age. But there are ways to use a slice of time on a routine basis that can help modify vascular risk. The body consists of interlinked systems that tend to self-repair and to seek the goal of normal function. Such a complex system is subject to the influence of training. We know that mastering tasks of dexterity, for example, playing the piano, requires repetition. In similar fashion, the cardiovascular system can be modified by training in the form of regular and sufficient exercise.

The cardiovascular system's responsiveness can be easily measured by subjecting it to stress. One form that has been studied is the cold pressor test. In this test, a person's hand is placed under ice water for a period of 2 minutes and then the blood pressure is measured. Generally the blood pressure increases sharply as a reaction to this stress. However, some of us react more sharply than others in that the blood pressure goes up very quickly. How quickly, and how quickly it comes down again, are useful predictors of vascular risk. These sharp reactors also react in the same fashion to any other sort of cardiovascular stress – as if the world is able to punish our bodies with our complicity.

Our response to stress can be modified by several means. Meditation has been shown to reduce stress responses. People who practice meditation often experience significantly lowered heart rates and blood pressures. The dramatic ability of our thoughts to modify cardiovascular behavior also suggests that the topics we spend time thinking about are important. Fuming while waiting in traffic increases blood pressure; exercising patience while waiting lowers it.

While ability to use one's thoughts as a health strategy may be a skill that all possess, some utilize it more than others. There may be a learning dimension to this as well so that skill, practice and proper guidance permit one to become more expert with such an intervention. For example, contemplation may have more benefit if it includes a focus pursuing inner goals. Actively choosing to commit time for meditation or contemplation may also confer a benefit since it demonstrates a measure of control over life's struggles. It is as if we are not only reacting, but are proactively choosing strategies for healthy living.

Another way to achieve cardiovascular benefits is by exercise. Some believe there is a "dose response" to exercise – if a little bit has some benefit, more exercise has greater benefit. Often we experience plateaus, where further efforts produce little additional benefit. Each of us can examine our own dose/response curve and choose activities accordingly. Regular exercise does appear to confer more benefit than occasional exercise. One concept underlying the use of exercise is that while rest is essential, a regular program of activity is always favored.

A specific example of the benefit of action has been demonstrated in patients who have narrowed arteries in their leg muscles. Since these arteries are in the periphery (that is away from the heart and brain), such narrowings are called peripheral arterial disease. These narrowings are from hardening of the arteries. At a certain amount of narrowing, blood flow through these vessels is restricted.

When we exercise our legs, we increase the demand for oxygen by the muscles. This increased oxygen demand requires an increase in the circulation – a cardiovascular response. Treatment for such narrowing vessels is dilatation or opening the blockages by using balloons – a process called angioplasty. High pressures are required in order to crack the plaque that is present in the blood vessels and to enlarge their diameter. Balloon angioplasty procedures are commonly performed in the United States on leg arteries.

An informative study of these treatments compared one group of patients who underwent balloon angioplasty to an equal number of subjects who followed a program of exercise. The group receiving the balloon angioplasty experienced an immediate increase in the blood flow to their legs. However, the group that followed exercise alone was able to walk further. One might have thought that increased blood flow would be accompanied by an increase in exercise ability. But the opposite was the case.

To receive a benefit from increased blood flow we have to train. To increase our exercise ability we have to exercise. As time passed in this study, gradual arterial restriction recurred in the balloon-treated arteries. After 3 years there was no difference in the amount of blood flow in the treated or the untreated group. However, at each and every point over the 3 years, the group that followed the exercise program was able to walk further than the group that was given the balloon intervention. The fact that a program of exercise provided a more powerful treatment benefit than balloon angioplasty confirms the power of physical activity.

This study also shows that the benefit of an uncommon and inexpensive intervention (exercise) used regularly is a positive contrast to a common, expensive one (balloon angioplasty). It is not very high tech to propose that the fundamental program for treatment of blocked leg arteries should include a program of regular exercise. And this low-tech solution is very cost effective.

The benefits of exercise are not only restricted to the leg arteries. Benefit is seen in any group of blood vessels that have blockages due to hardening of the arteries. As we have previously discussed, such blockages are in all of the blood vessels and in most all of us. So if you can't carve out time to meditate, you should dedicate some time for a program of regular exercise. Get some sneakers and use them.

Summary

- Stop or never start smoking.
- Consider using meditation for stress reduction. In its simplest form, helpful breathing exercises can be done using this pattern: breathe in slowly and, on the out breath, release the stressful thought.
- Exercise.

5   ATHEROSCLEROSIS +

As plaque builds up, there is easy access for bad cholesterol (LDL) in the blood to enter through the lining cells of the blood vessels and gain entrance to the plaque. Just as LDL can go into plaque, so it can also diffuse out again. LDL can be removed from plaque by lowering LDL in the bloodstream.

When the plaque is removed surgically or cracked by balloon angioplasty, the walls of the blood vessel have to be reconstituted. If these treatments resulted in a completely cleaned out vessel, then great durability would be expected. However, the man-made blood vessel wall does not last as long as the original one.

Since clamps are used to control bleeding when the blood vessel is opened, scarring can occur at focal points in the blood vessel wall. After angioplasty the blood vessel can become severely narrowed in as little as 90 days due to a scar-type process taking place. Such narrowing can occur in 30–40% of patients who undergo either surgery or balloon treatment (see Figures 5.1, 5.2).

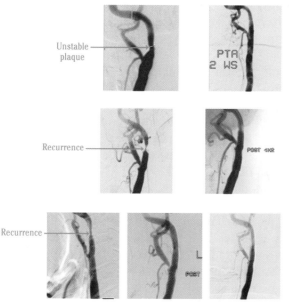

Figure 5.1
Top left: Unstable plaque causing a stroke in December 1996.
Top right: Improved blood flow after angioplasty and stent (flexible tube) insertion in January 1997.
Middle left: 5 months later, in June 1997, narrowing has recurred.
Middle right: improved blood flow after angioplasty.
Bottom left: 5 months later, in November 1997, blockage has recurred.
Centre bottom: Improved blood flow after angioplasty and further stent insertion.
Bottom right: 8 months later, in July 1998, blockage has recurred.

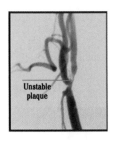 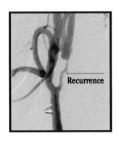

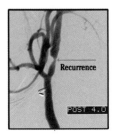 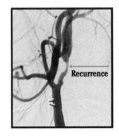

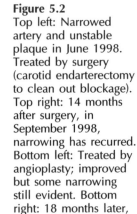

Figure 5.2
Top left: Narrowed artery and unstable plaque in June 1998. Treated by surgery (carotid endarterectomy to clean out blockage). Top right: 14 months after surgery, in September 1998, narrowing has recurred. Bottom left: Treated by angioplasty; improved but some narrowing still evident. Bottom right: 18 months later, in March 2001, narrowing has worsened.

The rapid tempo of the narrowing implies that it is not due to build-up of LDL or any forms of cholesterol. The process is really a type of scarring where the blood vessel is responding to a vascular injury. We call this process **atherosclerosis +**.

The new narrowing may have a different clinical fate than the original narrowing since there are not necessarily components of plaque involved. Recurrent narrowing after surgery or ballooning is more common than problems resulting from any original narrowing due to plaque. Scarring does not carry the same risk as an unstable plaque that is similarly narrow. Yet as this scarring process continues, such severe narrowing can occur that blood flow over the scar is restricted, causing symptoms to recur. The scar is tougher than plaque and is harder to stretch or crack by the use of balloons. There is often little LDL within the scar, which usually consists of various cells.

Current treatments aimed at modifying the cellular elements' response to injury have included embedding medicated stents (flexible tubes that keep the blood vessels open) after the balloons are inflated. The medication is designed to gradually leak out from the stent in an attempt to suppress the growth of new cells. Radiation has been used to try to restrict such cell growth. Although these two approaches serve to delay matters, they rarely stop them completely.

More durable vascular procedures are needed to constrain growth of overall healthcare costs since all of us are aging and an increased number of procedures can be expected. Unless we find a means to make the increased number of procedures more durable, financing such a robust growth in volume will be problematic. If narrowing could be addressed by a single procedure, there would be significant cost reductions.

Treated plaque represents only the tip of the atherosclerosis iceberg. The "target" plaque is almost never the only plaque that is present. Post-procedure care must include a broad program of intervention. Regular exercise, smoking cessation and an ensemble of medications will be necessary to stabilize other plaques and to modify how the treated plaque/blood vessel heals. Plumbing-type procedures do not "fix" the problem of vascular disease though they generally do buy some time. However, their use also insures that a new condition, atherosclerosis +, will be an issue to deal with at the treatment site. Thus we have added to the list of problems by resorting to procedural medicine.

Summary

- Modification of the scarring process in blood vessels is difficult.
- Post-procedure care includes a combination of ensemble medication and personal initiatives.

6   COMBINATION THERAPY

Understanding the plaque events that cause a heart attack or stroke allows a design strategy for medically modifying those events. Once unstable plaque has been identified, a program of stabilization is in order. Such a program would address the plaque itself, circulating blood and parts of the circulation downstream from the plaque. The aim is threefold:

- to make the plaque less prone to rupture
- to stop circulating blood from clotting over the unstable plaque
- to increase oxygen delivery at the tissue level.

Ideally, a biochemical strategy could be developed that would cause plaque to regress or simply go away. Lacking such potent medications that would act like Drano®, we are left with a three-pronged approach.

To make the plaque less prone to rupture, there are several approaches. Blood pressure reduction reduces the stress over the plaque. Reducing the lipid content within the plaque (making it more stable) can be done by any means that lowers the circulating level of cholesterol in the bloodstream. Diet, exercise and medication are the main approaches to this challenge. The most potent medication program for reduction of cholesterol is the use of statins (these drugs reduce the amount of cholesterol that is produced in the liver, although they have no effect on any cholesterol that enters the blood from food). Statins can reduce the cholesterol by more than 50% and do so in a dose-dependent manner. The higher the dose of a statin the more cholesterol lowering occurs. While it is not known if there is greater benefit from very low cholesterol levels as opposed to just lower ones, over time guideline standards have suggested that lower is better. And the target levels in the guidelines have steadily gone lower and lower. Creating a more fibrous covering or cap over the plaque would enhance stability. Reducing inflammation within the plaque would also strengthen the cap. In the future, medication programs will be available to accomplish this.

Modifying the behavior of the blood passing over the activated plaque requires the use of blood thinners. When circulating blood comes into contact with a ruptured plaque, a cascade of interactions occurs which represent the beginnings of clot formation. Platelets, small cells that circulate in the blood and which have a lifetime of 10 days, are the first blood component involved in this process. Agents that modify the behavior of platelets are called antiplatelet agents, the most common being aspirin.

The effect of aspirin on the platelets is immediate and irreversible, preventing them from becoming activated or sticky. A common side effect of aspirin is to make bruising of the skin more manifest. This is because the inactivated platelets are unable to stop the bleeding into the skin that occurs after trauma. Another way to think about the bruising is that it shows that the aspirin is working. Since the circulating platelets last for 10 days, the effects of a single aspirin dose will last for 10 days also. This is why aspirin is often discontinued many days before elective procedures that pose a risk of bleeding.

While aspirin is an effective antiplatelet agent, not all its users receive benefit. To enhance its benefit, other medications are often added, creating a combination approach. Sometimes clopidogrel (trade name Plavix®) is added to generate a more profound or synergistic effect. Such a combination is called a "super aspirin." This program of aspirin together with clopidogrel has been shown to be more effective than aspirin alone. It is often used for heart attack treatment and prevention, stent placement, and ballooning without or with stenting followed by radiation for treatment of atherosclerosis +.

Sometimes aspirin is provided in a combination formulation such as sustained release dipyridamole (trade name Aggrenox®) or with pravastatin (trade name Pravagard®). These preparations have a fixed aspirin dosage, which makes dose adjustment impossible unless one adds supplemental aspirin. A reduction in the dose of aspirin would require a reduction in the ingredients of the other component(s) of the combination preparation as well. Such a reduction might reduce the benefit of taking the combination formulation.

It is very important NOT to take aspirin and ibuprofen together because the effect of aspirin on the platelet can be blocked if ibuprofen is also circulating in the bloodstream. Ibuprofen also has an antiplatelet effect – though it is temporary. During the time that ibuprofen is present within the platelet, aspirin is not able to perform its function of irreversibly eliminating the clotting effect of the platelets. The ibuprofen blocks the access of aspirin to its molecular target. So if ibuprofen is to be taken for other conditions, it should be taken hours away from the aspirin dose. If the two are used together, then the patient will receive only a temporary effect from the ibuprofen and no permanent effect from aspirin.

30

Planning when to take aspirin might also provide additional benefit. Many strokes occur at night so taking aspirin as close as possible to bedtime would inhibit more platelets. Reducing the numbers of platelets that could react with active plaque pretreats the heart attack or stroke.

To increase oxygen delivery downstream from the blockage, we need to enhance the ability of the body to break clots that form over the activated plaque, which is then swept away into the smaller arteries. Proteins that can dissolve clots are present in the lining cells of arteries. Medication such as statins can change the amount of these proteins and thus their effect. Another approach is to improve the ability of the arteries to enlarge themselves. The blood vessel wall has muscle cells within it and these cells can be made to either contract or relax. These muscle cells will relax when exposed to nitric oxide, increasing blood flow as the blood vessel enlarges. Nitric oxide is produced by the blood vessel's lining cells. The cholesterol-lowering statins also possess the ability to increase production of nitric oxide. This effect is completely separate from cholesterol lowering. The ability of the statins to produce this positive effect can be demonstrated in normal blood vessels after a week of medication use. Statins make normal blood vessels behave super-normally. If statin use is stopped, the effect is lost very quickly and there may be a rebound effect where the arteries are less able to relax. Such a rebound effect should lead to caution when planning elimination of cholesterol-lowering medication before surgical procedures. It is possible that these medications, in contrast to the blood thinners, should not be stopped before surgery.

Since the goal of medication is to reduce the chance of a heart attack or stroke, the most effective program is likely to be one that incorporates various drugs that are active at different locations in the plaque. Cancer chemotherapy uses much the same notion with the use of several agents in combination to optimize the effectiveness of each.

When several medications are used together, there can be interactions between the various agents that can prove harmful. Care must be taken when selecting drugs and timing their use. Effective use of combinations of drugs provides **pharmacologic insurance**, which lowers risk. Such a combination can limit the effect or size of a heart attack or stroke. Finally, it should be added that effective combinations might include non-prescription medication as well as prescription ones.

Summary

- Targets for combination therapy include the plaque, circulating blood and downstream or collateral blood flow.

- Plaque: diet, exercise, statins.
- Circulating blood: aspirin alone or in combination with clopidogrel (Plavix®) or sustained release dipyridiamole (Aggrenox®).
- Downstream: statins, exercise.
- Never take ibuprofen and aspirin at the same time.
- Aspirin might work best if taken at bedtime.

7 VITAMINS

Vitamins are chemicals that our bodies need for survival but which we do not produce. A lack of vitamins can produce disease. The lack of niacin produces pellagra, lack of vitamin C produces scurvy, while the lack of B12 produces pernicious anemia. The bodily functions that vitamins support range from making bones strong (vitamin D), providing vision (vitamin A), to producing blood-clotting proteins (vitamin K). Vitamins are classified as either water soluble (B and C) or fat soluble (A, D, E, K).

Most people on a balanced diet receive enough vitamins to avoid any deficiency. Foods are generally supplemented to provide adequate amounts of vitamins. The idea that taking an excessive or large amount of vitamins might have positive health consequences dates to the 1960s. Then Linus Pauling, who had won two Nobel prizes, proposed that high or mega doses of vitamin C would prevent the common cold. Many grams had to be ingested each day to provide this benefit. However, studies to prove his theory were negative. Unless sufficient water was taken with mega C, kidney or bladder stones could occur. So colds were not prevented and taking high-dose vitamin C could be risky.

There has been much speculation about vitamin E, which is an antioxidant. Though it is used to keep potato chips crisp, its benefit for humans has been elusive. In the United Kingdom, a study of vitamin E and the statin simvastatin (Zocor®) showed that the combination eliminated cardiovascular benefits. It is thought that vitamin E reduced the amount of good cholesterol (HDL). No benefit has been shown for taking vitamin E and bleeding in the brain can occur. So vitamin E has not proven to be a useful addition.

Folic acid, a B vitamin, has shown the greatest promise. High doses of folic acid (5 mg/day) have been shown to lower the risk of open spine, called spina bifida, when taken during conception and gestation. Folic acid is also known to lower the level of homocysteine, an amino acid in the blood. Studies have shown that high levels of homocysteine (> 12 µmol/L) are associated with a twofold risk of heart attacks. Use of 1 mg/day after coronary balloon angioplasty reduced recurrent narrowing (atherosclerosis +) by 50% in patients with homocysteine levels < 12 µmol/L. Modification of the healing process in the coronary arteries confirms the validity of biochemically changing scar formation. While folic acid is normally taken in doses of 400 µg/day, higher doses were needed for the scar-reducing effect.

Medication programs focused on plaque stabilization may therefore need to include folic acid. It is unknown whether there is benefit from taking folic acid PRIOR to experiencing activated plaque. However, folic acid remains a viable candidate as part of the combination therapy approach for modifying unstable plaque.

Summary

- Folic acid in augmented doses (perhaps 5 mg/day) may be the best vitamin for vascular health. You need to be sure that you are not deficient in B12 because, if so, taking folic acid without B12 shots would not be adequate.

8   HEART RHYTHM DISTURBANCES – ATRIAL FIBRILLATION

Case study 6

John, a 35-year-old songwriter and musician, had occasionally noted what he called a "subsonic vibration deep in my chest" which was not associated with any other symptoms. John compared the vibration to the feeling produced when "you step in front of an oncoming car and then get back on the sidewalk to keep from being hit." He had no light-headedness, dizziness, faintness or weakness. Since our hearts beat more than 100,000 times each day, most of us do not pay any attention to our heart rhythm and are unaware of it. John had no inkling of any trouble, other than the occasional "thrilling" that occurred. He "took it for granted that it was pounding away down there in regular time."

Early one morning while drinking coffee he noted a problem with his vision that had never occurred before. Very suddenly "the whole right side of vision went out on me." He ran to the bathroom mirror but was unable to recognize himself. Yet he had no weakness, paralysis, imbalance, numbness or tingling. In reality, John had suffered a stroke. A clot from his heart had traveled to the back of his brain, affecting his vision.

John had no family history of stroke and no personal history of high blood pressure, diabetes or smoking. He had no indication of blocked arteries, yet was now having a stroke that affected the vision to his right in both eyes. He did not have a tear in a normal artery that had caused the stroke; his stroke was caused by a heart rhythm disturbance called atrial fibrillation. This condition affects 2–3% of the entire population below 65 and more than 7% of those older than 65. It is the most common adult rhythm disturbance in the USA, affecting more than 10 million Americans, and is a common cause of stroke.

Most rhythm disturbances are felt at night, though they also occur during the day. Perhaps being away from the cares of the day enhances our awareness of our body's mechanical workings. Lying back against a firm mattress may also enhance the effect of a disturbed heart rhythm. Generally, atrial fibrillation produces no symptoms, though some will have a sudden sense of weakness or even faint. This rhythm disturbance generally causes a faster than normal and irregular heart beat. While it can occur with diseases of the heart valves (such as mitral valve narrowing from rheumatic fever) or from thyroid conditions, in most cases there is no identifiable cause.

When atrial fibrillation occurs, the collecting chambers of the heart do not contract normally. They actually quiver several times each second. These chambers normally collect blood that flows to the pumping (left-hand) side of the heart. About 20% of the heart's blood is collected when the upper chambers contract normally. When they do not, the work of the heart is reduced by 20%, which sometimes is noticeable. When the upper chambers are not contracting normally, blood collects or pools and does not flow normally into the lower chambers. The pooling of this blood is similar to the sloshing of a washing machine. Rather than passing through the heart normally, the blood becomes stagnant and can form blood clots. If these clots are then pumped out by the heart, they are likely to pass into the brain since it receives more than 20% of the heart's output. Such a traveling clot can produce an embolic stroke when it is eventually stopped by the progressively narrowing arteries in the brain.

Individuals with atrial fibrillation who are under age 65 have an annual stroke risk of 1% – IF there is no history of high blood pressure, diabetes, prior stroke or electrocardiogram (EKG) change. Persons above age 65 who have these risk factors, experience an annual risk of embolic stroke from atrial fibrillation of nearly 5%. These strokes generally occur without prior warnings and most often occur during the day.

People identified as having atrial fibrillation are placed on a medical program of anticoagulants to lower stroke risk. With few exceptions every patient with atrial fibrillation should be on a blood thinner unless there is an excessive risk of bleeding. For those below 65 without risk factors, aspirin is generally given. For those older than 65, anticoagulation with warfarin will lower stroke risk. An appropriate level of blood thinning with warfarin will reduce the risk of stroke from 5% to 1%, a more than 70% reduction! Newer medications called direct thrombin inhibitors are being tested to see if they are as effective as warfarin for atrial fibrillation. These new agents do not require periodic monitoring of the blood-thinning effect, which is needed with warfarin. Patients on these agents can eat foods that contain vitamin K, while those who take warfarin have to avoid such foods.

The downside to taking blood thinners is an increased risk of bleeding. Generally, the use of warfarin requires careful and periodic monitoring to prevent the medication from becoming too strong. Frequent blood testing is required to make sure that the effect of the medication is within the desired range. Low levels provide no protection and high levels produce an excessive risk of bleeding. The newer agents may prove to have a lower risk of hemorrhage than warfarin.

As many as 20% of all strokes that occur are due to atrial fibrillation and not from blocked arteries in the brain or in arteries that go to the brain. Yet most people who have atrial fibrillation, such as John, are unaware of their condition. Most who know of the condition are not taking blood thinners. The potential ability of certain drugs to prevent such a large number of strokes is ample reason for enhanced identification of this stroke-causing arrhythmia. Since so many millions of Americans have atrial fibrillation, we could prevent a large number of strokes each year by appropriate medical therapy. We should do this.

Summary

• All patients with atrial fibrillation need to take some form of anti-coagulation. For those younger than 65 with no other risk factors, aspirin is adequate. However, for those older than 65, adjusted dose warfarin (Coumadin®) reduces stroke risk from 5% per year to less than 1%. Careful monitoring is necessary to make warfarin use safer.

9   BAD SPELLS

Brief disturbances of normal functioning can be called "spells." The sudden shiver that occurs at times (reported by one as "a rabbit hopped over my grave") would be a spell. Spells can be caused by blocked heart arteries producing an episode of chest pain, or by a temporarily blocked brain artery producing symptoms of a TIA. Keys to unlocking the cause of a spell include careful consideration of the spell itself. Dr John H. Jackson, a famous nineteenth century British neurologist, said, "the study of the thing caused must precede the study of the cause of the thing." We could easily substitute the term "spell" for Jackson's "thing." Such a study is difficult when the "thing" that is affected is the reporter's own brain.

Case study 7

Jane had been traveling on business and was preparing a presentation to the board of directors of her company. She said:

> I was under a lot of stress and I was very tired. In the middle of the afternoon I had been speaking with a staff member and had difficulty getting words out. I wondered if I was making any sense. Later the staff person said that I was acting strangely. I got up to get some water as I felt somewhat nauseous and dizzy. After I got up, I walked back to the office. I remember looking into the office from the hallway, and I had a very strange feeling. I remember having an extremely uncomfortable sensation. Previously I had heard a person describe such an event as an "out of body experience" and I thought that is what it is all right.
>
> It was eerie and frightening. I had never felt anything like it before, yet I didn't stop and become frightened at that moment. I remember looking into the office from the hallway and having a strange feeling of watching a movie but with no pictures attached to it. As I continued to feel nauseous, I sat down on the top of the three steps that lead down to my office. I asked one of the staff members to fill my water glass. She got me the

water and apparently said to me "Should we call 911?" And this is the only part that I have no recollection of at all. She said that I said, "Yes." So they called 911, and my husband.

I said to everyone, "I'm fine, don't worry about me." Since I had a board meeting starting in 20 minutes, I stood up to go down these three steps to my office. Everyone was saying to me, "Don't move, we're worried about you." I sat down at my desk and was reassuring the others when I heard sirens. In short order paramedics filled my office and I said to them: "Where did you come from?" They answered they had been called about me! They asked if I wanted to be carried off to the hospital, and I said, "No, no, I feel fine." They took my blood pressure, which was very high and I said to them, "I'm exhausted, I'm under stress." With the blood pressure being up, it seemed to explain the whole thing. I did put it all together and said that I was OK; I could explain the whole thing. It all seemed very rational to me.

I probably would have not sought any medical help whatsoever afterwards. Everyone else said that I didn't totally black out, but there was that moment when I responded and didn't remember it later. But a physician who came to the board meeting told me that I needed to slow down and see my doctor.

After additional reflection about the episode, she was able to further refine the experience: "It happened so fleetingly. The first one was maybe 15 seconds and the second about 30 seconds. It was all so very fast. It is not the same as going to a frightful movie – I knew that something mental or physical must have been going on in me to cause it. The sensations were very distinct and not at all pleasurable. Eerie is the best word to describe the state."

Most of us have experienced the mental state called *déjà vu* – something new is experienced as something familiar in our past. Yogi Berra called it "*déjà vu* all over again." It is not known why such feelings occur, these feelings of familiarity, yet they are very common. However, most of us have not experienced the opposite of *déjà vu*. The opposite state, a sense of the familiar as strange or non-familiar, is called *jamais vu*. When told of the opposite of *déjà vu*, Jane responded: "Yes, yes that's it, because somehow that phrase best fits the sensation."

Her physician arranged for Jane to have a magnetic resonance imaging (MRI) brain scan. This showed what was read as a stroke involving the right side of the brain in the temporal lobe. Yet her symptoms seemed very different from the warning symptoms of stroke that were presented previously. She did not have weakness, paralysis, facial drawing, thick or absent speech, imbalance, double vision, or lack of vision. She had experienced a new thing in her spell. She had positive phenomena rather than the usual negative phenomena of a TIA. The sense of strangeness with familiar things, watching a movie without any pictures, and of not remembering orders that had been given are not TIA symptoms.

Her theory that the whole thing was a faint did not match the symptoms. She had never fainted before. If she had fainted it is unlikely that she could have given orders. When people faint upon immediately standing up, then they generally faint or go down again. Yet she had stood up and walked to her office without assistance. So her rationalizing or labeling the event was incorrect. The scan interpretation was also incorrect. The spell was not caused by a stroke, but by a brain tumor. Her spell was not a lack of oxygen due to a clogged artery or from a clot that traveled to the right side of the brain in the temporal lobe. Her event was an electrical one – a small seizure.

Jane's assessment of stress as the trigger may have been correct. Stress is well known to be a trigger in patients who have a seizure disorder or epilepsy. Seizures occur more frequently during stress. Lack of sleep, out of town travel, the pressure of a board presentation were all additive. It is important to recognize the importance of stress as a trigger, not a cause. Diagnostic medicine is often impaired or clouded when stress is used to form the basis of the clinical hypothesis. All concerned would have to agree that there was a great deal of stress in Jane's life at that point. Yet to have dismissed the event by labeling it as due only to stress would have been incorrect. It is very important to consider stress when deciding on medical management but not for diagnostic decisions.

Jane's case was made more complicated by the incorrect scan reading, which suggested therapy for a condition she did not have. Her symptoms did not fit the classic mold for a TIA. The fact that the scan was abnormal in the temporal region suggested that the symptoms were being caused by something there. Since the symptoms were not those associated with stroke, there must be something else present that was causing the intermittent symptoms. When symptoms do not fit a diagnostic condition, but are very different, alternative clinical hypotheses must be considered.

We must be informed medical consumers, aware of stroke warning symptoms and the appropriate action to follow. We must be very informed consumers to make sure that a medical answer has the correct "fit." Perhaps the first thing that we are told may be reasonable, but that does not mean it is correct. Knowing more about the nature of spells helps each of us refine our judgment about their cause. Knowledge can bring power – the power to know what is the accurate cause.

Negative spells may be a TIA, but positive ones are probably something else. In Jane's case, the spell was not a TIA, it was something worse. Her spells were transient tumor attacks. That an event or spell may be brief and the person may seem normal shortly thereafter does not mean that nothing important has happened. When something very new and very different occurs, urgent investigation is in order. Taking an aspirin and dismissing the spell as stress is not a wise thing to do. Stress can and may be the trigger, but it is surely NOT the cause. Knowing the cause may change your life – as it did for Jane.

Summary

- All medical explanations are theories and need to be discarded when they no longer fit the clinical condition.
- Stress can trigger things, but there is a cause underneath – which should always be sought.

10   PERIPHERAL ARTERY DISEASE

Hardening of the arteries occurs in all blood vessels, including those that go to the lower extremities. When blockages occur in these arteries, the condition is called peripheral arterial disease (PAD), which affects 8–12 million Americans. Symptoms such as weakness and cramping in the legs occur because insufficient oxygen is delivered to the muscles in the legs. This condition is known as claudication. When enough blockage exists to limit flow, symptoms are very reproducible with the same level of exertion.

A very similar symptom occurs when the spine is markedly narrow. Narrowing in the spine may cause back pain, but once more the primary symptom is a reduction of exercise capability. People with spinal narrowing have good days and bad days, but those with vascular narrowing do not have such variability in symptoms with exercise.

By the time symptoms of claudication occur in the legs, the blockages must be very severe. When a patient's blockages are sufficient to restrict blood flow at rest, the individual is at risk of losing the leg due to gangrene. This condition is called critical limb ischemia. However, the blocking process is present many decades before symptoms are generated, so this condition is generally without symptoms, although no less important. Only about 10% of patients with PAD have classic symptoms of claudication, so most patients do not know they have blockages in their leg arteries.

Testing can easily detect such blockages. Usually the blood pressure in the leg arteries is greater than that in the arm arteries. It is possible to measure the pressure in the arms and legs and produce a ratio which is called the ankle:brachial index (abbreviated ABI). Since the ankle pressure is greater than the arm pressure, the ABI is normally greater than 1. When this number falls below 1, then there is blockage in the in-flow arteries to the legs. When the number is less than 0.5, the blockage is severe.

Hardening of the arteries in the legs is a severe problem. The 5-year average survival of those with ABIs below 0.5 is worse than the 5-year survival rate for patients with lung cancer. The reason hardening of the arteries in the legs is so serious is that these blockages usually indicate advanced blockages in other arteries in the body. The risk of a heart attack in a PAD patient is similar to that of cardiac patients even when the PAD patient has no cardiac symptoms. Early detection of PAD is essential since it indicates narrowing in other parts of the body. Recognition of the process, on-going hardening of the arteries, might be a catalyst to change behavior which can lower vascular risk.

Exercise is the cornerstone of treatment for blocked leg arteries. The importance of exercise was shown in a study of patients who underwent balloon treatment of the blockage compared to a group that did not receive such treatment. For those who received treatment there was an immediate increase in the amount of blood flowing in the previously narrowed artery. However, the group who did not receive balloon treatment was consistently able to walk further than their balloon-treated counterparts. After several years there was recurrent narrowing in the treated group so their blood flow was again reduced. But at every point for 5 years the non-treated group was still out-walking those who had received balloon treatment.

"Slickers", such as pentoxifylline (Trental®) or cilostazol (Pletal®) are medications used to make the blood flow more freely and they provide some relief of rest symptoms in patients with severe disease. But these medications make no difference to the eventual outcome of PAD, since the problem is hardening of the arteries. Whether an ensemble approach of drug combinations will provide further benefit to patients with PAD has yet to be proven. But if the process is the same in all arteries, then it makes sense that more aggressive medical treatment may be helpful.

Infrequent use of ultrasound screening for detecting PAD in patients without symptoms reduces the opportunity for early intervention even though these studies are easy to perform. This non-invasive test should be part of a general vascular assessment and could be performed on a serial basis to document evidence of change. One could even imagine using the study to gauge therapy and perhaps even guide it.

PAD is a risk factor for heart disease, and when present, strongly suggests that aggressive treatment measures are warranted. Yet patients with PAD receive less treatment than cardiac patients. PAD is markedly under-recognized by most physicians. So all of us as patients need to know about it. Knowledge brings power – the power to change.

Summary

- Get your peripheral arteries studied with an ABI (ankle:brachial index).
- The cardiac risk of PAD patients is similar to that of patients who have had a heart attack, even when the PAD patient has no cardiac symptoms.

11 ANGIOLOGY – THE STUDY OF BLOOD VESSELS

Vascular care in the USA is best characterized as a "Fire Department" model. You have a problem, call 911, and arrive at the emergency department. There you are triaged to the best group to put a fire extinguisher on the problem – putting out the vascular fire. At discharge from hospital, there is less than a 50/50 chance that you will receive the ensemble of medications that might prevent you from having to return in the next 60 days. In parts of the USA the use of aspirin after a stroke when patients are discharged from hospital is as low as 36%. What you don't take can't help you.

The United States has the highest use rates of complex medical equipment and the highest volume of vascular procedures in the world. Plainly, such frequent use of costly equipment is very expensive. In the United States more of the gross national product is spent on healthcare than any other country. Since the USA has the world's largest economy, that translates into the world's greatest healthcare expenditure – 1.7 trillion dollars each year. Since vascular events increase with age, it can be expected that demand for such services will increase in the United States and in all western societies. Continuing the current program of vascular care will necessitate an even greater flow of dollars into medical care.

In a study of outpatient medicine conducted by phone interviews and review of medical records, the majority of Americans were not receiving the medications that were indicated for their conditions. Specifically, heart patients were being treated "better" than stroke patients but only by a small amount.

Compliance, whether patients actually take the medications that have been prescribed for them, is also a major issue. The average time that a patient takes a cholesterol-lowering statin after a heart attack is about 11 months. Such medication should probably be a component of long-term ensemble therapy. Benefits shown in studies of patients with manifest heart disease and stroke are often not received by most other patients. Usual care often means no or little care. A certain contributor to the high rate of vascular events in the United States is the lack of effective secondary prevention. All of us are stakeholders in the prevention and treatment of vascular disease.

Medical and surgical specialties developed historically around an anatomical model. We have different specialists for the arteries in our neck, brain, heart, abdomen, and legs. Some physicians perform surgery, some use catheters and some give medications. But we do not have specialists that concentrate on all of the arteries in the body. Such a specialty is known in European countries and is called angiology – literally study of the blood vessels. Another definition of angiology is integrated vascular care. Such a program is possible since the process of hardening of the arteries is the same in every blood vessel. Unstable plaque in a heart artery is the same as unstable plaque in a carotid artery or a brain artery. A common thread produces the clinical events that we know as heart attack or stroke and this common thread can be modified, IF identified.

What would such a specialty look like? Its focus should be prevention – since it is easier to prevent a stroke than to treat one. It would have as its central goal changing patient behavior, since patients have such great power based upon their choices. One way to modify behavior would be to show each patient what their arteries look like. Though seeing a chest x-ray of another patient with lung cancer makes little impact on the viewer, showing that viewer his/her own x-ray of lung cancer makes an enormous impact.

Current non-invasive technologies permit easy visualization of arteries by a variety of diagnostic means (see Figure 11.1). Yet most medical

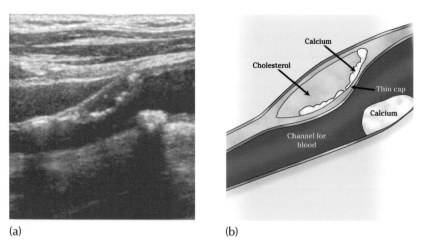

(a)   (b)

Figure 11.1 A carotid artery with unstable plaque. (a) Ultrasound image. Courtesy Henrik Sillesen. (b) Diagramatic representation.

insurance won't pay for these studies until the patient has a problem – hence the fire department model. So the angiologist must have access to this technology at a price that is easily affordable. Universal access is another worthwhile goal. Because vascular care is presently distributed among several different specialists, only those patients with a lot of free time can go and see all the necessary physicians.

Imaging of the arteries will be a crucial component of angiology care. Use and encouragement of lifestyle change will also be essential. Such efforts will enhance the benefit of the ensemble medication. There is great power in what we do as well as what we take.

The angiologist would try to stratify vascular risk: how much hardening of the arteries is present? Are those identified plaques "unstable"? If so, an aggressive program of medical intervention would be warranted. Were this program to fail, then a vascular procedure might be necessary to see if risk could be further reduced. One benefit of stratification would be a reduction in the number of procedures performed on an elective basis. Catheter laboratories and operating rooms would continue to be used for rescue, but diagnostic medicine could be conducted in a non-invasive setting. Angiology care might also enhance the durability of the various vascular procedures that are performed. This benefit might also impact the volume of procedures by reduction of repeat procedures.

The medical cornerstone of the angiologist's practice would be the use of ensemble medication on a long-term basis to prevent heart attacks and strokes. Choice of the best medical therapy would be guided by the results of well-conducted clinical trials, but aggressive combination therapies would probably provide the greatest benefit. Drug–drug interactions would be monitored as would potential side effects. Proper monitoring of the effects of medication would require periodic blood tests and probably imaging studies as well.

To create the angiology specialty might take as long as 7 years since medical students would need to be attracted to the field as an area of postgraduate training. The development of imaging skills during postgraduate training would have to be codified and refined. Yet how many of us would choose to wait as long as 7 years for mainstream medicine to respond to our vascular needs? We need angiologists today as well as tomorrow.

The stakeholders in integrated vascular care include patients and families as well as angiologists. All stakeholders share responsibility. If medicine is slow, then we can choose to act, even now. Knowing what the angiologist should do is not enough. Rather we need to know what we as patients should do and can do. The blueprint outlined in this text might serve as a guide or light for each of our paths. The coming revolution in vascular care – the creation of integrated vascular care – can be hastened by our learning and active participation. If the journey is long, START TODAY.

Summary

- TOGETHER we will create the next medical revolution: integrated care for our blood vessels. Such a program is called ANGIOLOGY.

12 CHAPTER SUMMARIES

Chapter 1: The problem

- Heart attacks and strokes occur when blockages in arteries become UNSTABLE, not just narrow.
- Most heart attacks occur in arteries that have only mild narrowing.
- It is important to know the nature of the narrowing in our arteries, not just how narrow.
- Unstable plaques create RISK which declines over time – this risk can be modified by medication and personal initiatives.
- Unstable plaque causes a heart attack or stroke when the plaque tears or dissects. Such tears can HEAL, as is known to occur with dissections in normal blood vessel walls.

Chapter 2: Cholesterol

- Cholesterol levels are only personally predictive when low or high. Mid-range values do not indicate whether you will have a heart attack or stroke.
- Cholesterol-lowering medications, the statins, reduce heart attack risk by means other than lowering cholesterol levels. The statins then have NON-CHOLESTEROL EFFECTS.

Chapter 3: Early warnings

- Angina is an early warning symptom of coronary insufficiency. It is defined as chest tightness or pressure, often with an ache in either arm (often the left) or jaw ache in concert with exertion.
- TIAs are warnings of an impending stroke. These sudden, tempo-rary and stereotypic spells (they are always the same) include diffi-culty speaking, imbalance, numbness to one side of the body (often face and arm or face/arm/leg), weakness to one side of the body (often face and arm or face/arm/leg), blindness in one eye, double vision. These generally last only 5 minutes or less.

Chapter 4: Reducing risk

- Stop or never start smoking.
- Consider using meditation for stress reduction. In its simplest form, helpful breathing exercises can be done using this pattern: breathe in slowly and, on the out breath, release the stressful thought.
- Exercise.

Chapter 5: Atherosclerosis +

- Modification of the scarring process in blood vessels is difficult.
- Post-procedure care includes combination medication and personal initiatives.

Chapter 6: Combination therapy

- Targets for combination therapy include the plaque, circulating blood and downstream or collateral blood flow.
- Plaque: diet, exercise, statins.
- Circulating blood: aspirin alone or in combination with clopidogrel (Plavix®) or sustained release dipyridiamole (Aggrenox®).
- Downstream: statins, exercise.
- Never take ibuprofen and aspirin at the same time.
- Aspirin might work best if taken at bedtime.

Chapter 7: Vitamins

- Folic acid in augmented doses (perhaps 5 mg/day) may be the best vitamin for vascular health. You need to be sure that you are not deficient in B12 because, if so, taking folic acid without B12 shots would not be adequate.

Chapter 8: Heart rhythm disturbances

- All patients with atrial fibrillation need to take some form of anti-coagulation. For those younger than 65 with no other risk factors, aspirin is adequate. However, for those older than 65, adjusted dose warfarin (Coumadin®) reduces stroke risk from 5% per year to less than 1%. Careful monitoring is necessary to make warfarin use safer.

Chapter 9: Bad spells

- All medical explanations are theories and need to be discarded when they no longer fit the clinical condition.
- Stress can trigger things, but there is a cause underneath – which should always be sought.

Chapter 10: Peripheral artery disease

- Get your peripheral arteries studied with an ABI (ankle:brachial index).
- The cardiac risk of PAD patients is similar to that of patients who have had a heart attack, even when the PAD patient has no cardiac symptoms.

Chapter 11: Angiology

- TOGETHER we will create the next medical revolution: integrated care for our blood vessels. Such a program is called ANGIOLOGY.

GLOSSARY OF TERMS

activated or "hot" plaque When hardening of the arteries, which produces plaque, becomes unstable then there is rupture of the contents of the plaque into the bloodstream. This produces clotting over the rupture site. At this point the plaque is considered to have become activated or "hot." Hot plaque produces heart attack and stroke.

angiogram An x-ray movie made by injecting dye into the body's arteries and then filming as the dye flows; literally a movie study of the blood vessels. A synonymous name is arteriogram. This is an invasive study – the body has to be entered with a catheter and various wires.

angiology The study of blood vessels and their diseases.

angioplasty Breaking plaque by means of balloon inflation. This technique is also called endovascular because it is taking place within the blood vessel. Often after ballooning, a metal sleeve or stent is placed to keep the artery open.

ankle:brachial index (ABI) The result of dividing the blood pressure in the ankle by the blood pressure in the arm (brachial). The fraction should be 1.0 or greater since the blood pressure is higher in the legs than the arms. A lower number means that there is some obstruction or blockage to the arteries in the legs.

atherosclerosis Literally hardening of the arteries due to the presence of fibrous tissue and calcium. The plaques that produce atherosclerotic narrowing are firm or hard.

atherosclerosis + The name given to recurrent blockages after balloon angioplasty and/or stenting. This is a scar process that is due to growth of muscle cells into the cracked segment of plaque.

atrial fibrillation A rapid heart rhythm where the collecting chambers (atria) are not synchronized with the pumping chamber (ventricle). The rapid quivering of the atria is called fibrillation. This is stroke-producing arrhythmia.

balloon angioplasty The opening of clogged blood vessels by inflating a balloon at great pressures just beneath the plaque.

CHD Synonymous with coronary artery disease (CAD). Coronary heart disease or coronary artery disease (CAD); blockages of the heart's blood vessels.

claudication Symptoms produced when too little blood flows to the leg muscles.

clot   Liquid blood that has become solid.

critical limb ischemia   Such severe blockages in the legs that loss of limb from gangrene is possible.

dissection   A tear in the inside lining of the blood vessel. Something that angioplasty may do when the balloon is inflated.

dizziness +   The combination of dizziness with double vision, facial numbness, thick speech, incoordination, and inability to walk.

hardening of the arteries   A colloquial name for atherosclerosis.

heart attack   Death of heart muscle when oxygen is not delivered due to blockage of a heart artery. Also known as acute coronary syndrome or ACS.

lipids   Fat. Various forms are cholesterol, triglyceride, low density lipoprotein (LDL), high density lipoprotein (HDL), very low density lipoprotein (VLDL).

peripheral arterial disease (PAD or sometimes called PVD)   Blockages of leg arteries by atherosclerosis.

plaque   The actual material in the blood vessel wall that comprises atherosclerotic changes. The plaque has a cap as well as inside materials.

plaque stabilization   An approach to try to keep plaque from becoming unstable; to keep plaque from rupturing. To keep plaque from continuing to grow and reduce the diameter of the blood vessel.

quiescent   Asymptomatic or stable plaque.

revascularization   Changing a blood vessel by surgical means (cleaning it out) or cracking a plaque (balloon angioplasty).

rupture   What happens when plaque becomes "hot." The cap or cover over the plaque is rent and so the contents of the plaque spill into the bloodstream.

statins   Cholesterol-lowering medications. Sometimes also known as reductase inhibitors.

stroke   The death of brain tissue when oxygen is not delivered due to a blockage of a brain artery or a bleed.

unstable plaque   Another term for "hot plaque." Plaque that is prone to rupture. Generally it has a thin fibrous cap.

vulnerable plaque   Synonymous with unstable plaque.

INDEX

Note: page numbers in *italics* refer to figures and tables